GW00499679

A Detailed Air Fryer Recipe Book

A Detailed Recipe Book with Delicious Recipes for keep on enjoying healthy meals and Get fit

Martine Haley

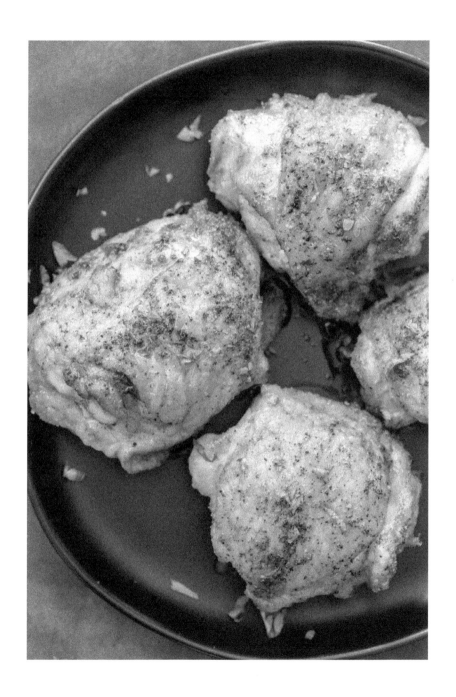

Table of Contents

© Copyright 2021 by Martine Haley - All rights reserved. The following Book is reproduced below with the goal of providing information that is as accurate and reliable as possible. Regardless, purchasing this Book can be seen as consent to the fact that both the publisher and the author of this book are in no way experts on the topics discussed within and that any recommendations or suggestions that are made herein are for entertainment purposes only. Professionals should be consulted as needed prior to undertaking any of the action endorsed herein. This declaration is deemed fair and valid by both the American Bar Association and the Committee of Publishers Association and is legally binding throughout the United States. Furthermore, the transmission, duplication, or reproduction of any of the following work including specific information will be considered an illegal act irrespective of if it is done electronically or in print. This extends to creating a secondary or tertiary copy of the work or a recorded copy and is only allowed with the express written consent from the Publisher. All additional right reserved. The information in the following pages is broadly considered a truthful and accurate account of facts and as such, any inattention, use, or misuse of the information in question by the reader will render any resulting actions solely under their purview. There are no scenarios in which the publisher or the original author of this work can be in any fashion deemed liable for any hardship or damages that may befall them after undertaking information described herein. Additionally, the information in the following pages is intended only for informational purposes and should thus be thought of as universal. As befitting its nature, it is presented without assurance regarding its prolonged validity or interim quality. Trademarks that are mentioned are done without written consent and can in no way be considered an endorsement from the trademark holder.

INTRODUCTION

An air fryer is a kitchen appliance designed to deliver a tasty, crispy, golden-brown morsel of food without the use of oil or other cooking fats. It uses hot air instead of oil or other cooking fats to cook food quickly and evenly.

The air fryer can be used for making fried chips in addition to other foods.

There are several varieties of air fryers. One of the main categories is made up of countertop air fryers designed for individual use in the kitchen. These models sit on the worktop or counter top and feature a basket that sits on a wire rack. This forms the base that holds hot air that cooks food as it passes through it.

air fryer's air fryers are designed to help you make healthy and filling meals. Our electric fryers are perfect for people who want fresh, homemade fries without all of the fat. Our air fryer features a light-weight aluminum design that lets you move the appliance from room to room without worry. Each air fryer is also equipped with a thermostat, making it easy to adjust the temperature as needed.

An air fryer is an appliance that cooks food using high-speed air circulation. It is a perfect alternative to deep frying, baking or roasting, and works great for cooking fast and healthy meals.

How Does an Air Fryer Work?

The fan draws warm air from the bottom of the chamber, which rises and cools as it circulates. The food is then placed in the middle of the basket, and the fan circulates air around it, cooking it all at once. Food cooks faster than if you fried it in oil or baked it in an oven. The food doesn't become soggy like fried food does, either. Because the air circulates around the food rather than through it, you can use much less oil in your Air Fryer. Best of all, since no oil is being used for cooking, there's much less of an environmental impact!

What Types of Air Fryers are Available?

Air fryers come in a variety of sizes as well as different colors and designs. You may find one that has a View Master-like chrome trim or one with a retro design pattern that blends easily into your décor. Some Air fryers are as small as a rice cooker while others can be used to make large batches of French fries with recipes you create on your tablet! Some Air Fryer models have "smart" features that allow you to cook multiple foods at the same time; others have timers so you can automatically set them for particular times during the day. All versions sterilize their own cooking plates by running them through a clean cycle between batches!

When you are looking for a new air fryer, you should take a look at air fryer Cookware. We have all of the features you are looking for in an air fryer, including built in racks that will allow you to cook a full size meal for your family. We also have a variety of accessories that will give you an even better cooking experience.

We are proud to introduce air fryer Cookware, the premier brand in air fryers. You can rest assured that we only use the best materials to ensure our products will work for years to come. Our air fryers feature built-in racks, so you can cook a full-size meal at once. They also include an adjustable thermostat that ranges from 120 to 500 degrees Fahrenheit.

Whether you are looking to impress your family with gourmet French fries or just want to make your favorite chicken drumsticks and vegetables, air fryer Cookware has everything you need. Every item has been carefully tested to ensure safe and responsible use. All of our products carry a One Year Limited Manufacturer Warranty, so you can be confident that they will serve your needs well.

Lemony Salmon

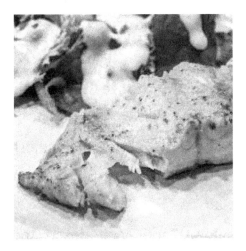

Basic Recipe

Preparation Time: 5 minutes

Cooking Time: 10 minutes

Serving: 2

Ingredients:

- 1 tbsp. offresh lemon juice
- ½ tbsp olive oil
- Salt and ground black pepper, as required
- 1 garlic clove, minced
- ½ tsp. fresh thyme leaves, chopped
- 2 (7-oz) Salmon fillets

Directions:

1. In a bowl, add all ingredients except the salmon and mix well. Add the salmon fillets and coat with the mixture generously.

2. Arrange the salmon fillets onto a lightly greased cooking rack, skin-side down. Arrange the drip pan in the bottom of the Instant Vortex Air Fryer Oven cooking chamber. Select "Air Fry" and then adjust the temperature to 400 °F. Set the time for 10 minutes and press "Start".

3. When the display shows "Add Food" insert the cooking rack in the bottom position. When the display shows "Turn Food" turn the fillets.

4. When the cooking time is complete, remove the tray from the Vortex Oven. Serve hot.

Nutrition: Calories 297 Carbs 0.8g Fat 15.8g Protein 38.7g

Miso Glazed Salmon

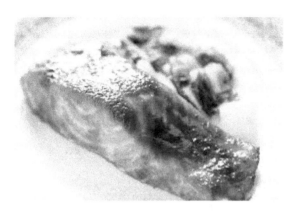

Basic Recipe

Preparation Time: 5 minutes

Cooking Time: 10 minutes

Serving: 4

Ingredients:

- 1/3 cup sake
- ¼ cup sugar
- ¼ cup red miso
- 1 tbsplow-sodium soy sauce
- 2 tbsp vegetable oil
- 4 (5-oz) Skinless salmon fillets, (1-inch thick)

Directions:

1. Place the sake, sugar, miso, soy sauce and oil into a bowl and beat until thoroughly combined. Rub the salmon fillets with the mixture generously. In a

plastic zip lock bag, place the salmon fillets with any remaining miso mixture.

2. Seal the bag and refrigerate to marinate for about 30 minutes Grease a baking dish that will fit in the Vortex Air Fryer Oven. Remove the salmon fillets from bag and shake off the excess marinade. Arrange the salmon fillets into the prepared baking dish.

    Arrange the drip pan in the bottom of the Instant Vortex Air Fryer Oven cooking chamber. Select "Broil" and Set the time for 5 minutes.

3. When the display shows "Add Food" insert the baking dish in the center position.

4. When the display shows "Turn Food" do not turn food. When cooking time is complete, remove the baking dish from the Vortex Oven. Serve hot.

Nutrition: Calories 335 Carbs 18.3g Fat 16.6g Protein 29.8g

Spiced Tilapia

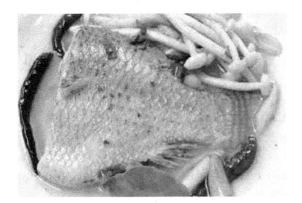

Basic Recipe

Preparation Time: 5 minutes

Cooking Time: 12 minutes

Serving: 2

Ingredients:

- ½ Tsplemon pepper seasoning
- ½ tsp. Garlic powder
- ½ tsp onion powder
- Salt and ground black pepper, as required
- 2 (6-oz) tilapia fillets
- 1 tbsp olive oil

Directions:

1. In a small bowl, mix together the spices, salt and black pepper. Coat the tilapia fillets with oil and then

rub with spice mixture. Arrange the tilapia fillets onto a lightly greased cooking rack, skin-side down.

2. Arrange the drip pan in the bottom of the Instant Vortex Air Fryer Oven cooking chamber. Select "Air Fry" and then adjust the temperature to 360 °F. Set the time for 12 minutes and press "Start".

3. When the display shows "Add Food" insert the cooking rack in the bottom position. When the display shows "Turn Food" turn the fillets.

4. When cooking time is complete, remove the tray from the Vortex Oven. Serve hot.

Nutrition: Calories 206 Carbs 0.2g Fat 8.6g Protein 31.9g

Crispy Tilapia

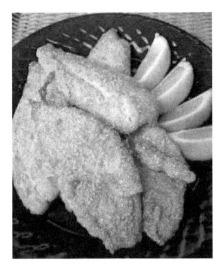

Basic Recipe

Preparation Time: 5 minutes

Cooking Time: 15 minutes

Serving: 2

Ingredients:

- ¾ cup cornflakes, crushed
- 1 (1-oz.) packet, dry ranch-style dressing mix
- 2½ tbsp vegetable oil
- 2eggs
- 4 (6-oz) tilapia fillets

Directions:

1. In a shallow bowl, beat the eggs. In another bowl, add the cornflakes, ranch dressing, and oil and mix

until a crumbly mixture form. Dip the fish fillets into egg and then, coat with the cornflake mixture.

2. Arrange the tilapia fillets onto the greased cooking tray. Arrange the drip pan in the bottom of the Instant Vortex Air Fryer Oven cooking chamber. Select "Air Fry" and then adjust the temperature to 355 °F. Set the time for 14 minutes and press "Start". When the display shows "Add Food" insert the cooking tray in the center position. When the display shows "Turn Food" turn the tilapia fillets. When cooking time is complete, remove the tray from the Vortex Oven. Serve hot.

Nutrition: Calories 291 Carbs 4.9g Fat 14.6g Protein 34.8g

Simple Haddock

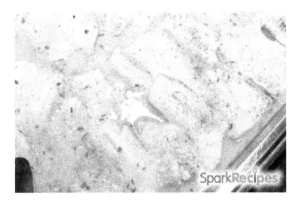

Basic Recipe

Preparation Time: 5 minutes

Cooking Time: 10 minutes

Serving: 2

Ingredients:

- 2 (6-oz) haddock fillets
- 1 tbsp olive oil
- Salt and ground black pepper, as required

Directions:

1. Coat the haddock fillets with oil and then, sprinkle with salt and black pepper. Arrange the haddock fillets onto a greased cooking rack and spray with cooking spray.

2. Arrange the drip pan in the bottom of the Instant Vortex Air Fryer Oven cooking chamber. Select "Air

Fry" and then adjust the temperature to 355 °F. Set the time for 8 minutes and press "Start".

3. When the display shows "Add Food" insert the cooking rack in the center position.

4. When the display shows "Turn Food" do not turn food.

5. When the cooking time is complete, remove the rack from the Vortex Oven. Serve hot.

Nutrition: Calories 251 Carbs 0g Fat 8.6g Protein 41.2g

Crispy Haddock

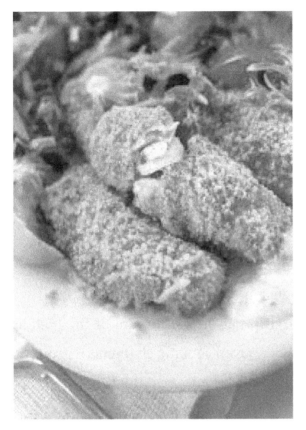

Basic Recipe

Preparation Time: 5 minutes

Cooking Time: 10 minutes

Serving: 3

Ingredients:

- ½ Cup flour
- ½ tsp. Paprika

- 1 egg, beaten
- ¼ cup mayonnaise
- 4 oz salt and vinegar potato chips, crushed finely
- 1 lb haddock fillet cut into 6 pieces

Direction:

1. In a shallow dish, mix together the flour and paprika. In a second shallow dish, add the egg and mayonnaise and beat well. In a third shallow dish, place the crushed potato chips.

2. Coat the fish pieces with flour mixture, then dip into egg mixture and finally coat with the potato chips. Arrange the fish pieces onto 2 cooking trays.

3. Arrange the drip pan in the bottom of the Instant Vortex Air Fryer Oven cooking chamber. Select "Air Fry" and then adjust the temperature to 370 °F. Set the time for 10 minutes and press "Start".

4. When the display shows "Add Food" insert 1 cooking tray in the top position and another in the bottom position.

5. When the display shows "Turn Food" do not turn the food but switch the position of cooking trays. When cooking time is complete, remove the trays from the Vortex Oven. Serve hot.

Nutrition: Calories 456 Carbs 40.9g Fat 22.7g Protein 43.5g

Vinegar Halibut

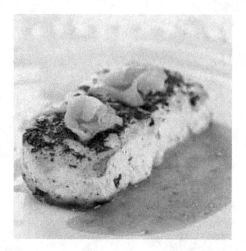

Basic Recipe

Preparation Time: 5 minutes

Cooking Time: 12 minutes

Serving: 2

Ingredients:

- 2 (5-oz) Halibut fillets
- 1 garlic cloves, minced
- 1 tsp fresh rosemary, minced
- 1 tbsp olive oil
- 1 tbsp red wine vinegar
- 1/8 tsp hot sauce

Directions:

1. In a large resealable bag, add all ingredients. Seal the bag and shale well to mix. Refrigerate to

marinate for at least 30 minutes Remove the fish fillets from the bag and shake off the excess marinade. Arrange the halibut fillets onto the greased cooking tray.

2. Arrange the drip pan in the bottom of the Instant Vortex Air Fryer Oven cooking chamber. Select "Bake" and then adjust the temperature to 450 °F. Set the time for 12 minutes and press "Start". When the display shows "Add Food" insert the cooking tray in the center position. When the display shows "Turn Food" turn the halibut fillets. When the cooking time is complete, remove the tray from the Vortex Oven. Serve hot.

Nutrition: Calories 223 Carbs 1g Fat 10.4g Protein 30g

Breaded Cod

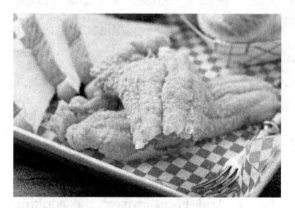

Basic Recipe

Preparation Time: 5 minutes

Cooking Time: 10 minutes

Serving: 4

Ingredients:

- 1/3 cup all-purpose flour
- Ground black pepper, as required
- 1 large egg
- 2 tbsp water
- 2/3 cup cornflakes, crushed
- 1 tbsp parmesan cheese, grated
- 1/8 tsp cayenne pepper
- 1 lb. Cod fillets –
- Salt, as required

Directions:

1. In a shallow dish, add the flour and black pepper and mix well. In a second shallow dish, add the egg and water and beat well. In a third shallow dish, add the cornflakes, cheese and cayenne pepper and mix well.

2. Season the cod fillets with salt evenly. Coat the fillets with flour mixture, then dip into egg mixture and finally coat with the cornflake mixture.

3. Arrange the cod fillets onto the greased cooking rack. Arrange the drip pan in the bottom of the Instant Vortex Air Fryer Oven cooking chamber. Select "Air Fry" and then adjust the temperature to 400 °F. Set the time for 10 minutes and press "Start".

4. When the display shows "Add Food" insert the cooking rack in the bottom position. When the display shows "Turn Food" turn the cod fillets. When cooking time is complete, remove the tray from the Vortex Oven. Serve hot.

Nutrition: Calories 168 Carbs 12.1g Fat 2.7g Protein 23.7g

Spicy Catfish

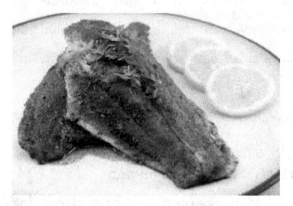

Basic Recipe

Preparation Time: 5 minutes

Cooking Time: 15 minutes

Serving: 4

Ingredients:

- 2 tbspcornmeal polenta
- 2 tsp cajun seasoning
- ½ tsp paprika
- ½ tsp garlic powder
- Salt, as required
- 2 (6-oz) catfish fillets
- 1 tbsp olive oil

Directions:

1. In a bowl, mix together the cornmeal, Cajun seasoning, paprika, garlic powder, and salt. Add the

catfish fillets and coat evenly with the mixture. Now, coat each fillet with oil.

2. Arrange the fish fillets onto a greased cooking rack and spray with cooking spray. Arrange the drip pan in the bottom of the Instant Vortex Air Fryer Oven cooking chamber. Select "Air Fry" and then adjust the temperature to 400 °F. Set the timer for 14 minutes and press "Start".

3. When the display shows "Add Food" insert the cooking rack in the center position. When the display shows "Turn Food" turn the fillets.

4. When cooking time is complete, remove the rack from the Vortex Oven. Serve hot.

Nutrition: Calories 32 Carbs 6.7g Fat 20.3g Protein 27.3g

Tuna Burgers

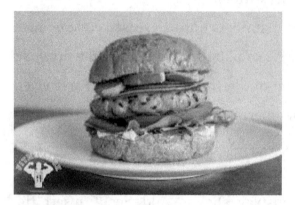

Basic Recipe

Preparation Time: 5 minutes

Cooking Time: 6 minutes

Serving: 4

Ingredients:

- 7 ozcanned tuna
- 1 large egg
- ¼ cup breadcrumbs
- 1 tbsp. Mustard
- ¼ tsp garlic powder
- ¼ tsp onion powder
- ¼ tspcayenne pepper
- Salt and ground black pepper, as required

Directions:

1. Add all the ingredients into a bowl and mix until well combined. Make 4 equal-sized patties from the mixture.

2. Arrange the patties onto a greased cooking rack. Arrange the drip pan in the bottom of the Instant Vortex Air Fryer Oven cooking chamber. Select "Air Fry" and then adjust the temperature to 400 °F. Set the time for 6 minutes and press "Start".

3. When the display shows "Add Food" insert the cooking rack in the center position.

4. When the display shows "Turn Food" turn the burgers.

5. When the cooking time is complete, remove the tray from the Vortex Oven. Serve hot.

Nutrition: Calories 151 Carbs 6.3g Fat 6.4g Protein 16.4g

Crispy Prawns

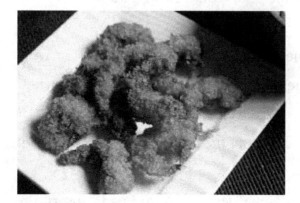

Basic Recipe

Preparation Time: 5 minutes

Cooking Time: 10 minutes

Serving: 4

Ingredients:

- 1egg
- ½ lb crushed nacho chips
- 12prawns, peeled and deveined

Directions:

1. In a shallow dish, beat the egg. In another shallow dish, place the crushed nacho chips. Coat the prawn into egg and then roll into nacho chips.

2. Arrange the coated prawns onto 2 cooking trays in a single layer. Arrange the drip pan in the bottom of the Instant Vortex Air Fryer Oven cooking chamber.

Select "Air Fry" and then adjust the temperature to 355 °F. Set the time for 8 minutes and press "Start".

3. When the display shows "Add Food" insert 1 tray in the top position and another in the bottom position. When the display shows "Turn Food" do not turn the food but switch the position of cooking trays. When cooking time is complete, remove the trays from the Vortex Oven. Serve hot.

Nutrition: Calories 386 Carbs 36.1g Fat 17g Protein 21g

Prawns in Butter Sauce

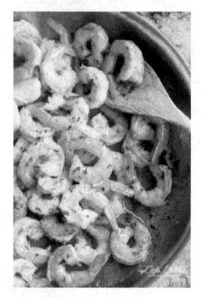

Basic Recipe

Preparation Time: 5 minutes

Cooking Time: 6 minutes

Serving: 2

Ingredients:

- ½ lb. Peeled and deveined large prawns

- 1 large garlic clove, minced

- 1 tbspbutter melted

- 1 tsp fresh lemon zest grated

Directions:

1. Add all the ingredients into a bowl and toss to coat well. Set aside at room temperature for about 30 minutes.

2. Arrange the prawn mixture into a baking dish that will fit in the Vortex Air Fryer Oven. Arrange the drip pan in the bottom of the Instant Vortex Air Fryer Oven cooking chamber. Select "Bake" and then adjust the temperature to 450 °F.

3. Set the time for 6 minutes and press "Start".

4. When the display shows "Add Food" insert the baking dish in the center position. When cooking time is complete, remove the baking dish from the Vortex Oven. When the display shows "Turn Food" do not turn food.

5. When cooking time is complete, remove the baking dish from the Vortex Oven. Serve hot.

Nutrition: Calories 189 Carbs 2.4g Fat 7.7g Protein 26g

Air Fried Chicken Tenderloin

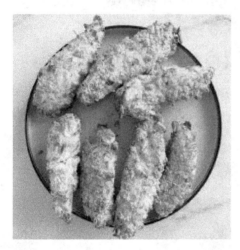

Basic Recipe

Preparation Time: 5 minutes

Cooking Time: 15 minutes

Serving: 8

Ingredients:

- ½ cup almond flour
- 1 egg, beaten
- 2 tablespoons coconut oil
- 8 chicken tenderloins
- Salt and pepper to taste

Directions:

1. Preheat the air fryer for 5 minutes Season the chicken tenderloin with salt and pepper to taste.

2. Soak in beaten eggs then dredge in almond flour. Place in the air fryer and brush with coconut oil.

3. Cook for 15 minutes at 375OF.

4. Halfway through the cooking time, give the fryer basket a shake to cook evenly.

Nutrition: Calories 130.3 Carbs 0.7g Protein 8.7 g Fat 10.3 g

Almond Flour Battered Chicken Cordon Bleu

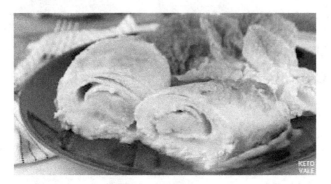

Basic Recipe

Preparation Time: 5 minutes

Cooking Time: 30 minutes

Serving: 2

Ingredients:

- ¼ cup almond flour
- 1 slice cheddar cheese
- 1 slice of ham
- 1 small egg, beaten
- 1 teaspoon parsley
- 2 chicken breasts, butterflied
- Salt and pepper to taste

Directions:

1. Season the chicken with parsley, salt and pepper to taste.
2. Place the cheese and ham in the middle of the chicken and roll. Secure with toothpick.
3. Soak the rolled-up chicken in egg and dredge in almond flour.
4. Place in the air fryer.
5. Cook for 30 minutes at 3500F.

Nutrition: Calories 1142 Carbs 5.5g Protein 79.4g Fat 89.1g

Almond Flour Coco-Milk Battered Chicken

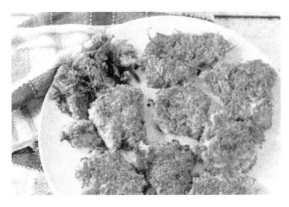

Basic Recipe

Preparation Time: 5 minutes

Cooking Time:30 minutes

Serving: 4

Ingredients:

- ¼ cup coconut milk
- ½ cup almond flour
- 1 ½ tablespoons old bay Cajun seasoning
- 1 egg, beaten
- 4 small chicken thighs
- Salt and pepper to taste

Directions:

1. Preheat the air fryer for 5 minutes
2. Mix the egg and coconut milk in a bowl.
3. Soak the chicken thighs in the beaten egg mixture.
4. In a mixing bowl, combine the almond flour, Cajun seasoning, salt and pepper.
5. Dredge the chicken thighs in the almond flour mixture.
6. Place in the air fryer basket.
7. Cook for 30 minutes at 3500F.

Nutrition:

Calories 590 Carbs3.2g Protein 32.5 g Fat 38.6g

Bacon 'n Egg-Substitute Bake

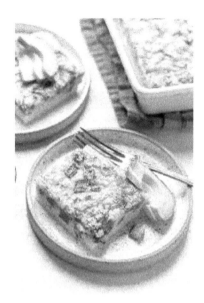

Basic Recipe

Preparation Time: 5 minutes

Cooking Time:30 minutes

Serving: 4

Ingredients:

- 1 (6 ounce) package Canadian bacon, quartered
- 1/2 cup 2% milk
- 1/4 teaspoon ground mustard
- 1/4 teaspoon salt
- 2 cups shredded Cheddar-Monterey Jack cheese blend

- 3/4 cup and 2 tablespoons egg substitute (such as Egg Beaters® Southwestern Style)
- 4 frozen hash brown patties

Directions:

1. Lightly grease baking pan of air fryer with cooking spray.
2. Evenly spread hash brown patties on bottom of pan. Top evenly with bacon and then followed by cheese.
3. In a bowl, whisk well mustard, salt, milk, and egg substitute. Pour over bacon mixture.
4. Cover air fryer baking pan with foil.
5. Preheat air fryer to 330oF.
6. Cook for another 20 minutes, remove foil and continue cooking for another 15 minutes or until eggs are set.
7. Serve and enjoy.

Nutrition: Calories 459 Carbs 21.0g Protein 29.4g Fat 28.5g

Baked Rice, Black Bean and Cheese

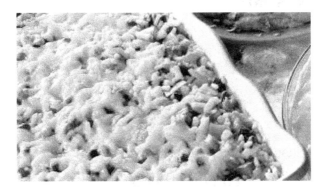

Intermediate Recipe

Preparation Time: 5 minutes

Cooking Time: 1 hour

Serving: 4

Ingredients:

- 1 cooked skinless boneless chicken breast halves, chopped
- 1 cup shredded Swiss cheese
- 1/2 (15 ounce) can black beans, Dry out
- 1/2 (4 ounce) can diced green chili peppers, Dry out
- 1/2 cup vegetable broth
- 1/2 medium zucchini, thinly sliced
- 1/4 cup sliced mushrooms
- 1/4 teaspoon cumin
- 1-1/2 teaspoons olive oil

- 2 tablespoons and 2 teaspoons diced onion
- 3 tablespoons brown rice
- 3 tablespoons shredded carrots
- Ground cayenne pepper to taste
- Salt to taste

Directions:

1. Lightly grease baking pan of air fryer with cooking spray. Add rice and broth. Cover pan with foil cook for 10 minutes at 390oF. Lower heat to 300oF and fluff rice. Cook for another 10 minutes Let it stand for 10 minutes and transfer to a bowl and set aside.

2. Add oil to same baking pan. Stir in onion and cook for 5 minutes at 330oF.

3. Stir in mushrooms, chicken, and zucchini. Mix well and cook for 5 minutes

4. Stir in cayenne pepper, salt, and cumin. Mix well and cook for another 2 minutes

5. Stir in ½ of the Swiss cheese, carrots, chilies, beans, and rice. Toss well to mix. Evenly spread in pan. Top with remaining cheese.

6. Cover pan with foil.

7. Cook for 15 minutes at 390oF and then remove foil and cook for another 5 to 10 minutes or until tops are lightly browned.

8. Serve and enjoy.

Nutrition: Calories 337 Carbs 11.5g Protein 25.3g Fat 21.0g

Basil-Garlic Breaded Chicken Bake

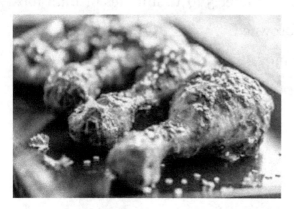

Intermediate Recipe

Preparation Time: 5 minutes

Cooking Time: 30 minutes

Serving: 2

Ingredients:

- 2 boneless skinless chicken breast halves (4 ounces each)
- 1 tablespoon butter, melted
- 1 large tomato, seeded and chopped
- 2 garlic cloves, minced
- 1 1/2 tablespoons minced fresh basil
- 1/2 tablespoon olive oil
- 1/2 teaspoon salt
- 1/4 cup all-purpose flour
- 1/4 cup egg substitute

- 1/4 cup grated Parmesan cheese
- 1/4 cup dry bread crumbs
- 1/4 teaspoon pepper

Directions:

1. In shallow bowl, whisk well egg substitute and place flour in a separate bowl. Dip chicken in flour, then egg, and then flour. In a small bowl whisk well the butter, bread crumbs and cheese. Sprinkle over chicken.

2. Lightly grease baking pan of air fryer with cooking spray. Place breaded chicken on bottom of pan. Cover with foil.

3. For 20 minutes, cook it on 390 F.

4. Meanwhile, in a bowl whisk well remaining ingredient.

5. Remove foil from pan and then pour over chicken the remaining Ingredients. Cook for 8 minutes. Serve and enjoy.

Nutrition: Calories 311 Carbs 22.0g Protein 31.0g Fat 11.0g

BBQ Chicken Recipe from Greece

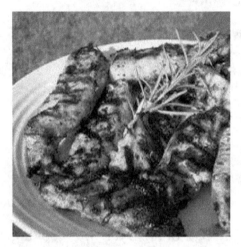

Basic Recipe

Preparation Time: 5 minutes

Cooking Time: 24minutes

Serving: 2

Ingredients:

- 1 (8 ounce) container fat-free plain yogurt
- 2 tablespoons fresh lemon juice
- 2 teaspoons dried oregano
- 1-pound skinless, boneless chicken breast halves - cut into 1-inch pieces
- 1 large red onion, cut into wedges
- 1/2 teaspoon lemon zest
- 1/2 teaspoon salt

- 1 large green bell pepper, cut into 1 1/2-inch pieces
- 1/3 cup crumbled feta cheese with basil and sun-dried tomatoes
- 1/4 teaspoon ground black pepper
- 1/4 teaspoon crushed dried rosemary

Directions:

1. In a shallow dish, mix well rosemary, pepper, salt, oregano, lemon juice, lemon zest, feta cheese, and yogurt. Add chicken and toss well to coat. Marinate in the ref for 3 hours.
2. Thread bell pepper, onion, and chicken pieces in skewers. Place on skewer rack.
3. For 12 minutes, cook it on 360oF. Turnover skewershalfway through cooking time. If needed, cook in batches.
4. Serve and enjoy.

Nutrition: Calories 242 Carbs 12.3g Protein 31.0g Fat 7.5g

BBQ Pineapple 'n Teriyaki Glazed Chicken

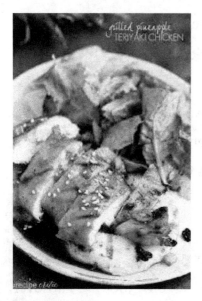

Basic Recipe

Preparation Time: 5 minutes

Cooking Time: 20 minutes

Serving: 2

Ingredients:

- ¼ cup pineapple juice
- ¼ teaspoon pepper
- ½ cup brown sugar
- ½ cup soy sauce
- ½ teaspoon salt

- 1 green bell pepper, cut into 1-inch cubes
- 1 red bell pepper, cut into 1-inch cubes
- 1 red onion, cut into 1-inch cubes
- 1 Tablespoon cornstarch
- 1 Tablespoon water
- 1 yellow red bell pepper, cut into 1-inch cubes
- 2 boneless skinless chicken breasts cut into 1-inch cubes
- 2 cups fresh pineapple cut into 1-inch cubes
- 2 garlic cloves, minced
- Green onions, for garnish

Directions:

1. In a saucepan, bring to a boil salt, pepper, garlic, pineapple juice, soy sauce, and brown sugar. In a small bowl whisk well, cornstarch and water. Slowly stir in to mixture in pan while whisking constantly. Simmer until thickened, around 3 minutes. Save ¼ cup of the sauce for basting and set aside.

2. In shallow dish, mix well chicken and remaining thickened sauce. Toss well to coat. Marinate in the ref for a half hour.

3. Thread bell pepper, onion, pineapple, and chicken pieces in skewers. Place on skewer rack in air fryer.

4. For 10 minutes, cook on 360oF. Turnover skewers halfway through cooking time. and baste with sauce. If needed, cook in batches.

5. Serve and enjoy with a sprinkle of green onions.

Nutrition: Calories 391 Carbs 58.7g Protein 31.2g Fat 3.4g

BBQ Turkey Meatballs with Cranberry Sauce

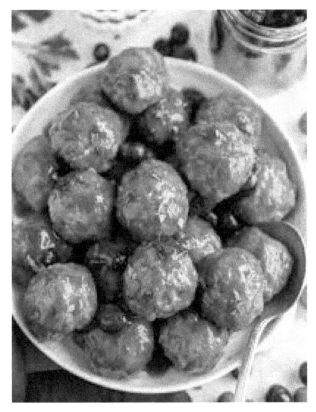

Basic Recipe

Preparation Time: 5 minutes

Cooking Time: 20 minutes

Serving: 4

Ingredients:

- 1 ½ tablespoons of water
- 2 teaspoons cider vinegar

- 1 tsp. salt and more to taste
- 1-pound ground turkey
- 1 1/2 tablespoons barbecue sauce
- 1/3 cup cranberry sauce
- 1/4-pound ground bacon

Directions:

1. In a bowl, mix well with hands the turkey, ground bacon and a tsp. of salt. Evenly form into 16 equal sized balls.

2. In a small saucepan boil cranberry sauce, barbecue sauce, water, cider vinegar, and a dash or two of salt. Mix well and simmer for 3 minutes

3. Thread meatballs in skewers and baste with cranberry sauce. Place on skewer rack in air fryer.

4. For 15 minutes, cook it on 360oF. Every after 5 minutes of cooking time, turnover skewers and baste with sauce. If needed, cook in batches.

5. Serve and enjoy.

Nutrition: Calories 217 Carbs 11.5g Protein 28.0g Fat 10.9g

Blueberry Overload French Toast

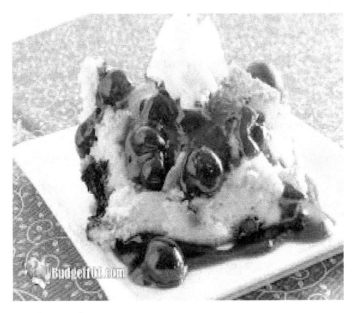

Basic Recipe

Preparation Time: 5 minutes

Cooking Time: 40minutes

Serving: 5

Ingredients:

- 1 (8 ounce) package cream cheese, cut into 1-inch cubes
- 1 cup fresh blueberries, divided
- 1 cup milk
- 1 tablespoon cornstarch
- 1/2 cup water

- 1/2 cup white sugar

- 1/2 teaspoon vanilla extract

- 1-1/2 teaspoons butter

- 2 tablespoons and 2 teaspoons maple syrup

- 6 eggs, beaten

- 6 slices day-old bread, cut into 1-inch cubes

Directions:

1. Lightly grease baking pan of air fryer with cooking spray.

2. Evenly spread half of the bread on bottom of pan. Sprinkle evenly the cream cheese and ½ cup blueberries. Add remaining bread on top.

3. In a large bowl, whisk well eggs, milk, syrup, and vanilla extract. Pour over bread mixture.

4. Cover air fryer baking pan with foil and refrigerate overnight.

5. Preheat air fryer to 330oF.

6. Cook for 25 minutes covered in foil, remove foil and cook for another 20 minutes or until middle is set.

7. Meanwhile, make the sauce by mixing cornstarch, water, and sugar in a saucepan and bring to a boil. Stir in remaining blueberries and simmer until thickened and blueberries have burst.

8. Serve and enjoy with blueberry syrup.

Nutrition: Calories 492 Carbs 51.9g Protein 15.1g Fat 24.8g

Broccoli-Rice 'n Cheese Casserole

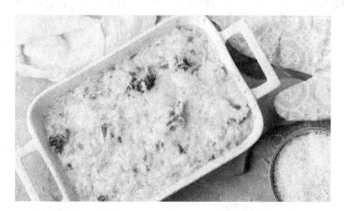

Basic Recipe

Preparation Time: 5 minutes

Cooking Time:30 minutes

Serving: 4

Ingredients:

- 1 (10 ounce) can chunk chicken, Dry out
- 1 cup uncooked instant rice
- 1 cup water
- 1/2 (10.75 ounce) can condensed cream of chicken soup
- 1/2 (10.75 ounce) can condensed cream of mushroom soup
- 1/2 cup milk
- 1/2 small white onion, chopped
- 1/2-pound processed cheese food

- 2 tablespoons butter
- 8-ounce frozen chopped broccoli

Directions:

1. Lightly grease baking pan of air fryer with cooking spray. Add water and bring to a boil at 390oF. Stir in rice and cook for 3 minutes.

2. Stir in processed cheese, onion, broccoli, milk, butter, chicken soup, mushroom soup, and chicken. Mix well. Cook for 15 minutes at 390oF, fluff mixture and continue cooking for another 10 minutes until tops are browned. Serve and enjoy.

Nutrition: Calories 752 Carbs 82.7g Protein 36.0g Fat 30.8g

Buffalo Style Chicken Dip

Basic Recipe

Preparation Time: 5 minutes

Cooking Time: 10 minutes

Serving: 4

Ingredients:

- 1 (8 ounce) package cream cheese, softened
- 1 tablespoon shredded pepper Jack cheese
- 1/2 pinch cayenne pepper, for garnish
- 1/2 pinch cayenne pepper, or to taste
- 1/4 cup and 2 tablespoons hot pepper sauce (such as Frank's Reshoot®)
- 1/4 cup blue cheese dressing
- 1/4 cup crumbled blue cheese
- 1/4 cup shredded pepper Jack cheese
- 1/4 teaspoon seafood seasoning (such as Old Bay®)
- 1-1/2 cups diced cooked rotisserie chicken

Directions:

1. Lightly grease baking pan of air fryer with cooking spray. Mix in cayenne pepper, seafood seasoning,

crumbled blue cheese, blue cheese dressing, pepper Jack, hot pepper sauce, cream cheese, and chicken.

2. For 15 minutes, cook it on 390 F.

3. Let it stand for 5 minutes and garnish with cayenne pepper.

4. Serve and enjoy.

Nutrition: Calories 405 Carbs 3.2g Protein 17.1g Fat 35.9g

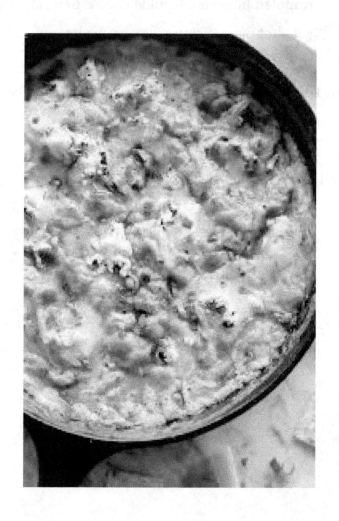

Buttered Spinach-Egg Omelet

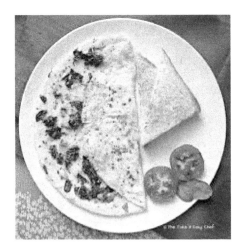

Basic Recipe

Preparation Time: 5 minutes

Cooking Time: 10 minutes

Serving: 4

Ingredients:

- ¼ cup coconut milk
- 1 tablespoon melted butter
- 1-pound baby spinach, chopped finely
- 3 tablespoons olive oil
- 4 eggs, beaten
- Salt and pepper to taste

Directions:

1. Preheat the air fryer for 5 minutes. In a mixing bowl, combine the eggs, coconut milk, olive oil, and butter until well-combined.

2. Add the spinach and season with salt and pepper to taste. Pour all ingredients in a baking dish that will fit in the air fryer. Bake at 3500F for 15 minutes

Nutrition: Calories 310 Carbs 3.6g Protein 13.6g Fat 26.8g

Caesar Marinated Grilled Chicken

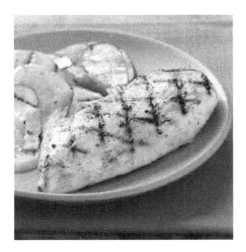

Basic Recipe

Preparation Time: 5 minutes

Cooking Time: 20 minutes

Serving: 3

Ingredients:

- ¼ cup crouton
- 1 teaspoon lemon zest. Form into ovals, skewer and grill.
- 1/2 cup Parmesan
- 1/4 cup breadcrumbs
- 1-pound ground chicken
- 2 tablespoons Caesar dressing and more for drizzling
- 2-4 romaine leaves

Directions:

1. In a shallow dish, mix well chicken, 2 tablespoons Caesar dressing, parmesan, and breadcrumbs. Mix well with hands. Form into 1-inch oval patties.

2. Thread chicken pieces in skewers. Place on skewer rack in air fryer.

3. For 12 minutes, cook it on 3600F. Turnover skewers halfway through cooking time. If needed, cook in batches.

4. Serve and enjoy on a bed of lettuce and sprinkle with croutons and extra dressing.

Nutrition: Calories 339 Carbs 9.5g Protein 32.6g Fat 18.9g

Cheese Stuffed Chicken

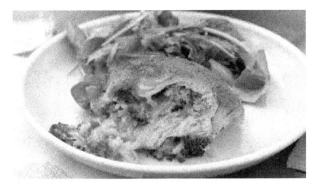

Basic Recipe

Preparation Time: 5 minutes

Cooking Time: 25 minutes

Serving: 4

Ingredients:

- 1 tablespoon creole seasoning
- 1 tablespoon olive oil
- 1 teaspoon garlic powder
- 1 teaspoon onion powder
- 4 chicken breasts, butterflied and pounded
- 4 slices Colby cheese
- 4 slices pepper jack cheese

Directions:

1. Preheat the air fryer to 3900F.
2. Place the grill pan accessory in the air fryer.

3. Create the dry rub by mixing in a bowl the creole seasoning, garlic powder, and onion powder. Season it with salt and pepper if desired.

4. Rub the seasoning on to the chicken.

5. Place the chicken on a working surface and place a slice each of pepper jack and Colby cheese.

6. Fold the chicken and secure the edges with toothpicks.

7. Brush chicken with olive oil.

8. Grill for 30 minutes and make sure to flip the meat every 10 minutes

Nutrition: Calories 727 Carbs 5.4 g Protein 73.1g Fat 45.9g

Cheeseburger Egg Rolls

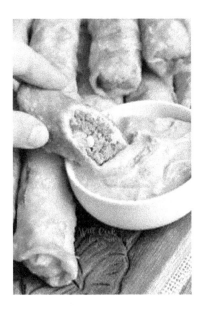

Basic Recipe

Preparation Time: 10 minutes

Cooking Time: 7 minutes

Servings: 6

Ingredients:

- 6 egg roll wrappers
- 6 chopped dill pickle chips
- 1 tbsp. yellow mustard
- 3 tbsp. cream cheese
- 3 tbsp. shredded cheddar cheese

- ½ C. chopped onion
- ½ C. chopped bell pepper
- ¼ tsp. onion powder
- ¼ tsp. garlic powder
- 8 ounces of raw lean ground beef

Directions:

1. In a skillet, add seasonings, beef, onion, and bell pepper. Stir and crumble beef till fully cooked, and vegetables are soft.
2. Take skillet off the heat and add cream cheese, mustard, and cheddar cheese, stirring till melted.
3. Pour beef mixture into a bowl and fold in pickles.
4. Lay out egg wrappers and place 1/6th of beef mixture into each one. Moisten egg roll wrapper edges with water. Fold sides to the middle and seal with water.
5. Repeat with all other egg rolls.
6. Place rolls into air fryer, one batch at a time.
7. Pour into the Oven rack/basket. Place the Rack on the middle-shelf of the Air Fryer Oven. Set temperature to 392°F, and set time to 7 minutes

Nutrition: Calories 153 Cal Fat 4 g Carbs 0 g Protein 12 g

Air Fried Grilled Steak

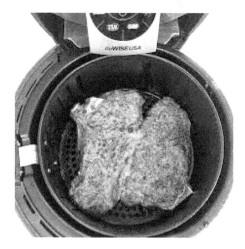

Basic Recipe

Preparation Time: 5 minutes

Cooking Time: 45 minutes

Servings: 2

Ingredients:

- 2 top sirloin steaks
- 3 tablespoons butter, melted
- 3 tablespoons olive oil
- Salt and pepper to taste

Directions:

1. Preheat the Air Fryer Oven for 5 minutes. Season the sirloin steaks with olive oil, salt and pepper.
2. Place the beef in the air fryer basket.
3. Cook for 45 minutes at 350°F.

---

4. Once cooked, serve with butter.

Nutrition: Calories 1536 Fat 123.7 g Carbs 0 g Protein 103.4 g

Juicy Cheeseburgers

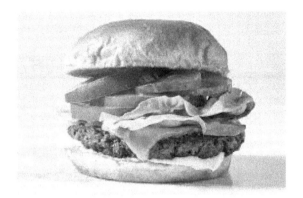

Basic Recipe

Preparation Time: 5 minutes

Cooking Time: 15 minutes

Servings: 4

Ingredients:

- 1 pound 93% lean ground beef
- 1 teaspoon Worcestershire sauce
- 1 tablespoon burger seasoning
- Salt
- Pepper
- Cooking oil
- 4 slices cheese
- Buns

Directions:

1. In a large bowl, mix the ground beef, Worcestershire, burger seasoning, and salt and pepper to taste until well blended. Spray the air fryer basket with cooking oil. You will need only a quick sprits. The burgers will produce oil as they cook. Shape the mixture into 4 patties. Place the burgers in the air fryer. The burgers should fit without the need to stack, but stacking is okay if necessary.

2. Pour into the Oven rack/basket. Place the Rack on the middle-shelf of the Air Fryer Oven. Set temperature to 375°F, and set time to 8 minutes Cook for 8 minutes Open the air fryer and flip the burgers. Cook for an additional 3 to 4 minutes Check the inside of the burgers to determine if they have finished cooking. You can stick a knife or fork in the center to examine the color.

3. Top each burger with a slice of cheese. Cook for an additional minute, or until the cheese has melted

4. Serve on buns with any additional toppings of your choice.

Nutrition: Calories 566 Cal Fat 39 g Carbs 0 g Protein 29 g

Spicy Thai Beef Stir-Fry

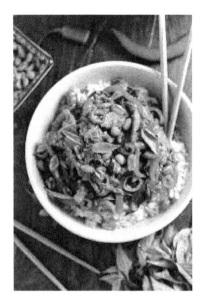

Basic Recipe

Preparation Time: 15 minutes

Cooking Time: 9 minutes

Servings: 4

Ingredients:

- 1-pound sirloin steaks, thinly sliced
- 2 tablespoons lime juice, divided
- ⅓Cup crunchy peanut butter
- ½ cup beef broth
- 1 tablespoon olive oil
- 1½ cups broccoli florets
- 2 cloves garlic, sliced

- 1 to 2 red chili peppers, sliced

Directions:

1. In a medium bowl, combine the steak with 1 tablespoon of the lime juice. Set aside.

2. Combine the peanut butter and beef broth in a small bowl and mix well. Dry out the beef and add the juice from the bowl into the peanut butter mixture.

3. In a 6-inch metal bowl, combine the olive oil, steak, and broccoli.

4. Pour into the Oven rack/basket. Place the Rack on the middle-shelf of the Air Fryer Oven. Set temperature to 375°F, and set time to 4 minutes Cook for 3 to 4 minutes or until the steak is almost cooked and the broccoli is crisp and tender, shaking the basket once during cooking time.

5. Add the garlic, chili peppers, and the peanut butter mixture and stir.

6. Cook for 3 to 5 minutes or until the sauce is bubbling and the broccoli is tender.

7. Serve over hot rice.

Nutrition: Calories 387 Cal Fat 22 g Carbs 0 g Protein 42 g

Beef Brisket Recipe from Texas

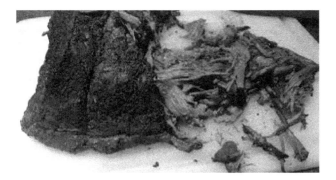

Basic Recipe

Preparation Time: 15 minutes

Cooking Time: 1 hour and 30 minutes

Servings: 8

Ingredients:

- 1 ½ cup beef stock
- 1 bay leaf
- 1 tablespoon garlic powder
- 1 tablespoon onion powder
- 2 pounds beef brisket, trimmed
- 2 tablespoons chili powder
- 2 teaspoons dry mustard
- 4 tablespoons olive oil
- Salt and pepper to taste

Directions:

1. Preheat the Air Fryer Oven for 5 minutes Place all ingredients in a deep baking dish that will fit in the air fryer.
2. Bake it for 1 hour and 30 minutes at 400°F.
3. Stir the beef every after 30 minutes to soak in the sauce.

Nutrition: Calories 306 Cal Fat 24.1 g Carbs 0 g Protein 18.3 g

Copycat Taco Bell Crunch Wraps

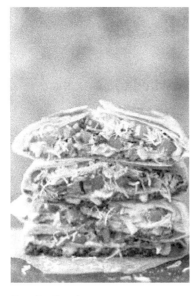

Basic Recipe

Preparation Time: 10 minutes

Cooking Time: 2 minutes

Servings: 6

Ingredients:

- 6 wheat tostadas
- 2 C. sour cream
- 2 C. Mexican blend cheese
- 2 C. shredded lettuce
- 12 ounces low-sodium nacho cheese
- 3 Roma tomatoes
- 6 12-inch wheat tortillas

- 1 1/3 C. water
- 2 packets low-sodium taco seasoning
- 2 pounds of lean ground beef

Directions:

1. Ensure your air fryer is preheated to 400 degrees.
2. Make beef according to taco seasoning packets.
3. Place 2/3 C. prepared beef, 4 tbsp. cheese, 1 tostada, 1/3 C. sour cream, 1/3 C. lettuce, 1/6th of tomatoes and 1/3 C. cheese on each tortilla.
4. Fold up tortillas edges and repeat with remaining ingredients.
5. Lay the folded sides of tortillas down into the air fryer and spray with olive oil.
6. Set temperature to 400°F, and set time to 2 minutes Cook 2 minutes till browned.

Nutrition: Calories 311 Cal Fat 9 g Carbs 0 g Protein 22 g

Air Fryer Beef Casserole

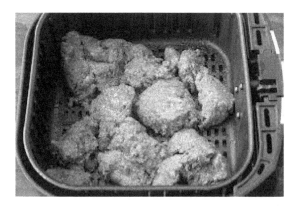

Basic Recipe

Preparation Time: 5 minutes

Cooking Time: 30 minutes

Servings: 4

Ingredients:

- 1 green bell pepper, seeded and chopped
- 1 onion, chopped
- 1-pound ground beef
- 3 cloves of garlic, minced
- 3 tablespoons olive oil
- 6 cups eggs, beaten
- Salt and pepper to taste

Directions:

1. Preheat the Air Fryer Oven for 5 minutes

2. In a baking dish that will fit in the air fryer, mix the ground beef, onion, garlic, olive oil, and bell pepper. Season it with salt and pepper to taste.

3. Pour in the beaten eggs and give a good stir.

4. Place the dish with the beef and egg mixture in the air fryer.

5. Pour into the Oven rack/basket. Place the Rack on the middle-shelf of the Air Fryer Oven. Set temperature to 325°F, and set time to 30 minutes. Bake it for 30 minutes

Nutrition:

Calories 1520 Cal Fat 125.11 g Carbs 0 g Protein 87.9 g

Meat Lovers' Pizza

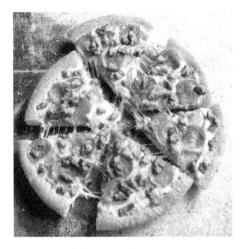

Intermediate Recipe

Preparation Time: 10 minutes

Cooking Time: 12 minutes

Servings: 2

Ingredients:

- 1 pre-prepared 7-inch pizza pie crust, defrosted if necessary
- 1/3 cup of marinara sauce
- 2 ounces of grilled steak, sliced into bite-sized pieces
- 2 ounces of salami, sliced fine
- 2 ounces of pepperoni, sliced fine
- ¼ cup of American cheese
- ¼ cup of shredded mozzarella cheese

Directions:

1. Preheat the Air Fryer Oven to 350 degrees. Lay the pizza dough flat on a sheet of parchment paper or tin foil, cut large enough to hold the entire pie crust, but small enough that it will leave the edges of the air frying basket uncovered to allow for air circulation. Using a fork, stab the pizza dough several times across the surface – piercing the pie crust will allow air to circulate throughout the crust and ensure even cooking. With a deep soup spoon, ladle the marinara sauce onto the pizza dough, and spread evenly in expanding circles over the surface of the pie-crust. Be sure to leave at least ½ inch of bare dough around the edges, to ensure that extra-crispy crunchy first bite of the crust! Distribute the pieces of steak and the slices of salami and pepperoni evenly over the sauce-covered dough, then sprinkle the cheese in an even layer on top.

2. Set the air fryer timer to 12 minutes, and place the pizza with foil or paper on the fryer's basket surface. Again, be sure to leave the edges of the basket uncovered to allow for proper air circulation, and don't let your bare fingers touch the hot surface. After 12 minutes, when the Air Fryer Oven shuts off, the cheese should be perfectly melted and lightly

crisped, and the pie crust should be golden brown. Using a spatula – or two, if necessary, remove the pizza from the air fryer basket and set on a serving plate. Wait a few minutes until the pie is cool enough to handle, then cut into slices and serve.

Nutrition: Calories 390 Cal Fat 21 g Carbs 34 g Fiber 3 g

Chimichurri Skirt Steak

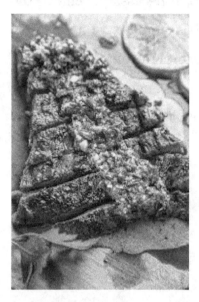

Basic Recipe

Preparation Time: 10 minutes

Cooking Time: 8 minutes

Servings: 2

Ingredients:

- 2 x 8 oz. skirt steak
- 1 cup finely chopped parsley
- ¼ cup finely chopped mint
- 2 tbsp. fresh oregano (washed & finely chopped)
- 3 finely chopped cloves of garlic
- 1 tsp. red pepper flakes (crushed)
- 1 tbsp. ground cumin

- 1 tsp. cayenne pepper
- 2 tsp. smoked paprika
- 1 tsp. salt
- ¼ tsp. pepper
- ¾ cup oil
- 3 tbsp. red wine vinegar

Directions:

1. Throw all the ingredients in a bowl (besides the steak) and mix well.
2. Put ¼ cup of the mixture in a plastic baggie with the steak and leave in the fridge overnight (2–24hrs).
3. Leave the bag out at room temperature for at least 30 min before popping into the air fryer. Preheat for a minute or two to 390° F before cooking until med–rare (8–10 min). Pour into the Oven rack/basket. Place the Rack on the middle-shelf of the Air Fryer Oven. Set temperature to 390°F, and set time to 10 minutes
4. Put 2 Tbsp. of the chimichurri mix on top of each steak before serving.

Nutrition: Calories 308.6 Cal Fat 22.6 g Carbs 3 g Protein 23.7 g

Country Fried Steak

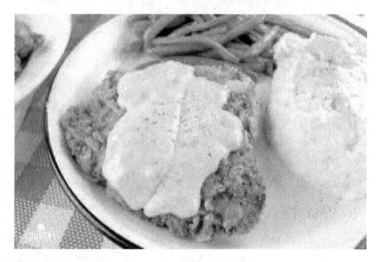

Basic Recipe

Preparation Time: 5 minutes

Cooking Time: 12 minutes

Servings: 2

Ingredients:

- 1 tsp. pepper
- 2 C. almond milk
- 2 tbsp. almond flour
- 6 ounces ground sausage meat
- 1 tsp. pepper
- 1 tsp. salt
- 1 tsp. garlic powder
- 1 tsp. onion powder

- 1 C. panko breadcrumbs
- 1 C. almond flour
- 3 beaten eggs
- 6 ounces sirloin steak, pounded till thin

Directions:

1. Season panko breadcrumbs with spices
2. Dredge steak in flour, then egg, and then seasoned panko mixture.
3. Place into air fryer basket.
4. Set temperature to 370°F, and set time to 12 minutes
5. To make sausage gravy, cook sausage and Dry outof fat, but reserve 2 tablespoons.
6. Add flour to sausage and mix until incorporated. Gradually mix in milk over medium to high heat till it becomes thick.
7. Season mixture with pepper and cook 3 minutes longer.
8. Serve steak topped with gravy and enjoy.

Nutrition: Calories 395 Cal Fat 11 g Carbs 0 g Protein 39 g

Creamy Burger & Potato Bake

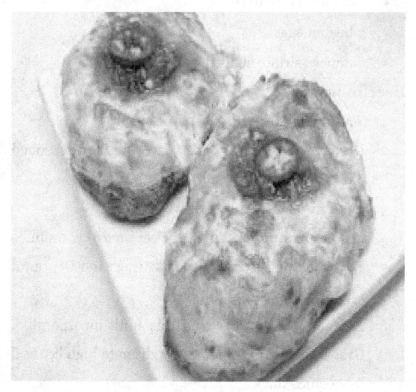

Intermediate Recipe

Preparation Time: 5 minutes

Cooking Time: 55 minutes

Servings: 3

Ingredients:

- Salt to taste

- Freshly ground pepper, to taste

- 1/2 (10.75 ounce) can condensed cream of mushroom soup

- 1/2-pound lean ground beef
- 1-1/2 cups peeled and thinly sliced potatoes
- 1/2 cup shredded Cheddar cheese
- 1/4 cup chopped onion
- 1/4 cup and 2 tablespoons milk

Directions:

1. Lightly grease baking pan of air fryer with cooking spray. Add ground beef. For 10 minutes, cook on 360°F
2. Stir and crumble halfway through cooking time.
3. Meanwhile, in a bowl, whisk well pepper, salt, milk, onion, and mushroom soup. Mix well.
4. Dry out fat off ground beef and transfer beef to a plate.
5. In same air fryer baking pan, layer ½ of potatoes on bottom, then ½ of soup mixture, and then ½ of beef. Repeat process.
6. Cover pan with foil.
7. Cook for 30 minutes Remove foil and cook for another 15 minutes or until potatoes are tender.
8. Serve and enjoy.

Nutrition: Calories 399 Cal Fat 26.9 g Carbs 0 g Protein 22.1 g

Beefy 'n Cheesy Spanish Rice Casserole

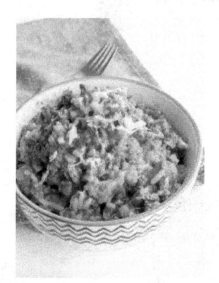

Intermediate Recipe

Preparation Time: 10 minutes

Cooking Time: 50 minutes

Servings: 3

Ingredients:

- 2 tablespoons chopped green bell pepper
- 1 tablespoon chopped fresh cilantro
- 1/2-pound lean ground beef
- 1/2 cup water
- 1/2 teaspoon salt
- 1/2 teaspoon brown sugar

- 1/2 pinch ground black pepper
- 1/3 cup uncooked long grain rice
- 1/4 cup finely chopped onion
- 1/4 cup chili sauce
- 1/4 teaspoon ground cumin
- 1/4 teaspoon Worcestershire sauce
- 1/4 cup shredded Cheddar cheese
- 1/2 (14.5 ounce) can canned tomatoes

Directions:

1. Lightly grease baking pan of air fryer with cooking spray. Add ground beef.
2. For 10 minutes, cook on 360°F Halfway through cooking time, stir and crumble beef. Discard excess fat,
3. Stir in pepper, Worcestershire sauce, cumin, brown sugar, salt, chili sauce, rice, water, tomatoes, green bell pepper, and onion. Mix well. Cover pan with foil and cook for 25 minutes. Stirring occasionally
4. Give it one last good stir, press down firmly and sprinkle cheese on top.
5. Cook uncovered for 15 minutes at 390°F until tops are lightly browned.
6. Serve and enjoy with chopped cilantro.

Nutrition: Calories 346 Cal Fat 19.1 g Carbs 0 g Protein 18.5 g

MAINS

Pumpkin and Pork Escallops

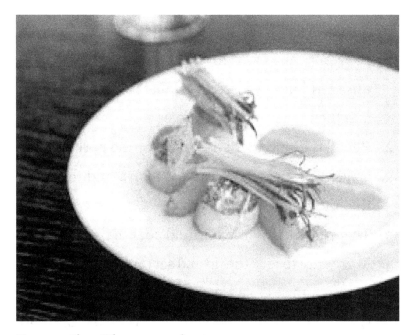

Preparation Time: 10 minutes

Cooking Time: 40 minutes

Servings: 4

Ingredients:

- 40 oz pork, ground
- 1 medium-sized pumpkin, cut into eighths
- 4 tbsp. dried sage
- 2 tbsp. clarified and unsalted butter

- 2 teaspoons dried thyme
- 2 teaspoons ground cinnamon
- 1 cup of fish broth
- 1 teaspoon of salt
- 1 teaspoon pepper

Directions:

1. Fix your Air fryer to sauté mode and melt the unsalted butter or use the skillet to melt the butter and then pour in your Air fryer.

2. Put all the spices in a bowl. Flavor the pork with the spices mix. Form the pork escallops. Add them into the Air fryer.

3. Then, add in the pumpkin and pour in the fish broth.

4. Make sure to lock the lid and set on a HIGH pressure for 40 minutes.

5. Quick-release the pressure and transfer the pork escallops to a plate.

6. Combine the pumpkin with the pork escallops and ladle up the sauce (if any) all over the meat.

Nutrition: Calories – 254 Protein – 57 g. Fat – 63 g. Carbs – 199 g.

Pork Curry with Cheese

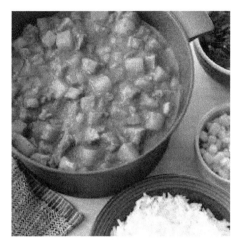

Preparation Time: 15 minutes

Cooking Time: 40 minutes

Servings: 4

Ingredients:

- 20 oz pork, cubed
- 1 cup of champignons, sliced up
- 1 cup of Parmesan cheese, grated
- 1 medium onion, peeled and chopped
- 2 garlic cloves, minced
- 1 green chili, seeded and diced
- 1 tablespoon ginger
- ½ a tablespoon turmeric
- 1 cup of vegetable stock

- 3 tablespoons red curry paste
- 2 teaspoons salt
- 1 teaspoon cumin
- ½ teaspoon curry powder
- ¼ teaspoon ground fenugreek
- ¼ teaspoon black pepper
- 1 tablespoon tomato paste
- 3 tablespoons freshly squeezed lemon juice
- 1 cup of spinach, chopped

Directions:

1. Set the pot to sauté mode and add the champignons to the inner pot to cook for 10 minutes.
2. Add in the onion and mix well, cook until clear and caramelized.
3. Add the chili, garlic, ginger, turmeric and sauté for 1-2 minutes.
4. Add all the remaining ingredients and cancel the sauté mode.
5. Be sure to cover the lid and cook on a HIGH pressure for around 40 minutes.
6. Naturally release the pressure.
7. Stir in the tomato paste, spinach and lemon juice.

8. Portion the curry into four bowls or mugs and dollop each bowl with the grated Parmesan cheese.

Nutrition: Calories – 247 Protein – 35 g. Fat – 45 g. Carbs – 213 g.

Lemon and Pork Chops in Tomato Sauce

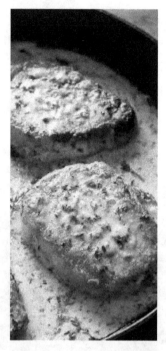

Preparation Time: 15 minutes

Cooking Time: 45 minutes

Servings: 3

Ingredients:

- 5 pieces 2-inch pork
- 1 cup of tomato sauce
- 1 lemon, diced
- 4 ounces pancetta, diced
- 2 teaspoons pepper

- 2 carrots, peeled and chopped
- 1 orange peeled and diced
- 1 medium shallot, chopped
- 1 tablespoon lemon zest, minced
- 3 teaspoons dried rosemary
- 4 teaspoons garlic, minced
- ½ cup of lemon juice
- ¼ cup of chicken broth
- soy sauce, to taste

Directions:

1. In a bowl, combine the pepper, lemon zest, dried rosemary and garlic. Toss the pork in the spices mix and pour the lemon juice over the meat. Then set the pork aside to marinate it for a couple of hours at room temperature or place in the fridge overnight.

2. Put all ingredients in your Air fryer and close the lid to let them cook on a HIGH pressure for about 45 minutes.

3. Release the pressure quickly and transfer the chops to a carving board.

4. Slice up the meat into strips. Divide into three plates and pour the soy sauce on top to serve.

Nutrition: Calories – 382 Protein – 74 g. Fat – 80 g. Carbs – 284 g.

Buckwheat with Pork Chunks

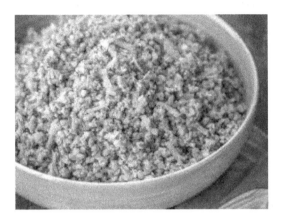

Preparation Time: 10 minutes

Cooking Time: 30 minutes

Servings: 4

Ingredients:

- 28 oz (1 can) pork chunks with broth, canned
- 1 cup of buckwheat, rinsed
- 4 medium onions, peeled and sliced
- 3 cups of water
- ½ teaspoon salt and pepper

Directions:

1. Immerse the buckwheat in the warm water for around 10 minutes. Then add in the buckwheat to your pot.

2. In a skillet or wok, fry the onions for 10 minutes until clear and caramelized. In a bowl, mash the pork using a fork.

3. Combine the buckwheat, pork chunks and caramelized onions and add to your Air fryer.

4. Make sure to lock the lid and cook on a HIGH pressure for 20 minutes.

5. Naturally release the pressure over 10 minutes.

6. Portion the buckwheat and pork chunks into four deep containers and dollop each bowl with the salt and pepper. Serve the buckwheat porridge and pork chunks with the coffee.

Nutrition: Calories – 285 Protein – 52 g. Fat – 79 g. Carbs – 237 g.

Lime Pork with Pineapple and Peanuts

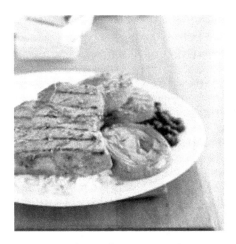

Preparation Time: 10 minutes

Cooking Time: 45 minutes

Servings: 4

Ingredients:

- 20 oz pork
- 1 cup of pineapple, diced
- 1 cup of peanuts
- 2 tablespoons soy sauce
- 1 tablespoon dry basil
- 5 garlic cloves, minced
- 4 tablespoons olive oil
- Salt as needed

- 4 tablespoons freshly squeezed lime juice
- ½ tablespoon of corn starch
- ½ cup of water

Directions:

1. Marinate the pork in the salt, soy sauce, dry basil, minced garlic and lime juice for at least few hours at room temperature or place in the fridge overnight.

2. Preheat the oven to 240°-260°F and roast the peanuts in the oven for 10 minutes until crispy and then let it cool completely. Then grind the peanuts using a food processor or blender.

3. Add the marinated pork and all the listed ingredients to your Air fryer.

4. Make sure to lock the lid and set the timer to 45 minutes and cook the pork on a MEAT/STEW mode.

5. Naturally release the pressure over 10 minutes.

6. Portion the pork into four deep containers and dollop each bowl with the salt and pepper. Serve the pork with the tea.

Nutrition: Calories – 374 Protein – 62 g. Fat – 72 g. Carbs – 271 g.

Pork in Tomato Sauce with Pineapple

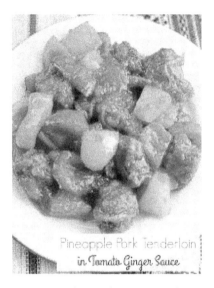

Pineapple Pork Tenderloin in Tomato Ginger Sauce

Preparation Time: 15 minutes

Cooking Time: 55 minutes

Servings: 3

Ingredients:

- 5 pieces 2-inch pork
- 1 cup of pineapple, cubed
- 1 cup of tomato sauce
- 4 ounces pancetta, diced
- 2 teaspoons pepper
- 2 carrots, peeled and chopped
- 3 teaspoons dried rosemary
- 4 teaspoons garlic, minced

- ½ cup of orange juice
- ¼ cup of chicken broth
- soy sauce, to taste

Directions:

1. Combine the pepper, dried rosemary and garlicin a bowl. Toss the pork in the spices mix. Then set the pork aside to marinate it for at least few hours or place in the fridge overnight.

2. Put all ingredients to your Air fryer and secure the lid to let itcook for about 55 minutes on a HIGH pressure.

3. Release the pressure quickly and transfer the pork to a carving board.

4. Slice up the meat into strips. Divide into three plates and pour the soy sauce on top to serve.

Nutrition: Calories – 382 Protein – 74 g. Fat – 82 g. Carbs – 286 g.

Pork in Tomato Sauce with Butter

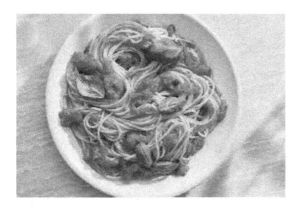

Preparation Time: 15 minutes

Cooking Time: 45 minutes

Servings: 4

Ingredients:

- 5 pieces 2-inch pork
- 1 cup of tomato sauce
- 4 tablespoons salted butter
- 5 garlic cloves, minced
- 3 teaspoons dried rosemary
- 2 teaspoons black pepper
- 1 teaspoon nutmeg
- 1 cup of chicken broth

Directions:

1. In a bowl, mix the dried rosemary, nutmeg, black pepper, and garlic. Toss the pork in the spices mix.

Then set the pork aside to marinate it for a couple of hours at room temperature or place in the fridge overnight.

2. Put all the ingredients in your Air fryer and close the lid to let them cook on a HIGH pressure for about 45 minutes.

3. Release the pressure and place the pork to a carving board.

4. Slice up the meat into strips and then divide into four bowls or plates and ladle up the tomato sauce and then spoon some salted butter on top to serve with the white bread and wine.

Nutrition: Calories – 393 Protein – 89 g. Fat – 92 g. Carbs – 293 g.

Pork with Lemon

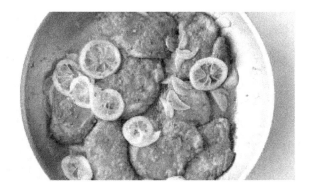

Preparation Time: 10 minutes

Cooking Time: 45 minutes

Servings: 3

Ingredients:

- 20 oz pork
- 2 lemons, peeled and diced
- 5 tablespoons liquid honey
- 2 tablespoon Gouda cheese, grated
- 2 tablespoons soy sauce
- 1 tablespoon dry basil
- 5 garlic cloves, minced
- 4 tablespoons olive oil
- Salt as needed
- 1 cup of freshly squeezed lemon juice
- ½ tablespoon of corn starch

- ½ cup of water

Directions:

1. Marinate the pork in the salt, soy sauce, dry basil, minced garlic, lemon juice and honey for a couple of hours at room temperature or place in the fridge overnight. Add the marinated pork and all other ingredients to your Air fryer.

2. Secure the lid, fix the timer to 45 minutes and cook the pork on MEAT/STEW option.

3. Naturally release the pressure for 10 minutes.

4. Serve and enjoy!

Nutrition: Calories – 379 Protein – 64 g. Fat – 74 g. Carbs – 277 g.

Spicy Pork Shoulder with Brown Rice

Preparation Time: 10 minute

Cooking Time: 65 minutes

Servings: 4

Ingredients:

- 1 cup of brown rice
- 30 oz pork shoulder, cut into half
- 1 tablespoon liquid smoke
- 5 tablespoons sunflower oil
- 1 cup of water
- 2 teaspoons chili pepper powder
- salt and pepper to taste
- brown rice or steamed green beans for serving (optional)

Directions:

1. Wash the brown rice several times and let the water boil to cook the rice for about 20 minutes. Add 2 tablespoons sunflower oil when the rice is ready.

2. Fix your Air fryer to sauté mode and pour some oil to heat it up.

3. Add in the pork, salt, chili pepper powder and pepper, brown each side for 5 minutes until the both sides are slightly browned. Transfer them to a plate.

4. Put the water and liquid smoke to the Air fryer and place the meat and spoon the rice.

5. Make sure to lock the lid and cook for60 minutes on a HIGH pressure, release pressure naturally over 10 minutes.

6. Transfer the pork meat to the cutting board and shred using 2 forks. Portion the pork into four plates and dollop each plate with the cooking liquid. Serve it with the rice or green beans on the side.

Nutrition: Calories – 384 Protein – 64 g. Fat – 75 g. Carbs – 275 g.

Pork Ribs with Honey

Preparation Time: 10 minutes

Cooking Time: 50 minutes

Servings: 3

Ingredients:

- 15 oz pork back ribs
- 2 tablespoons honey
- 1 teaspoon sesame oil
- 2 tablespoons oyster sauce
- 1 teaspoon salt
- 1 teaspoon sugar
- 1 cup of water
- ½ cup of liquid smoke

Directions:

1. In a bowl, marinate the pork back ribs in honey. Then set the meat aside to marinate for a couple of hours at room temperature or place in the fridge overnight.
2. Add all the listed ingredients to the Air fryer.
3. Make sure to lock the lid and cook on MEAT/STEW mode for 50 minutes.
4. Naturally release the pressure over 10 minutes.

5. Portion the pork ribs into three plates and dollop each plate with the cooking liquid and oyster sauce. Serve it with the buckwheat or brown rice on the side if you prefer.

Nutrition: Calories – 364 Protein – 76 g. Fat – 70 g. Carbs – 264 g.

Sausages Omelet with Bread and Peanuts

Preparation Time: 10 minutes

Cooking Time: 35 minutes

Servings: 4

Ingredients:

- 8 eggs
- 25 oz smoked pork sausages, sliced
- 1 cup of peanuts
- 25 oz bread, diced
- 2 tablespoons olive oil
- 2 medium carrots, peeled and diced
- 1 medium onion, peeled and chopped
- salt and black pepper, to taste
- 1 bunch of parsley

Directions:

1. Whisk the eggs using an electric hand mixer until there is a creamy consistency and homogenous mass.

2. In a frying pan or wok, warm up the olive oil and fry the bread for 10 minutes until golden brown and

crispy. Then add in the sausages and chopped onion and fry for 5-10 minutes until clear and caramelized.

3. Mix the eggs with the salt, pepper, salmon, bread and onion in a bowl, and whisk them well.

4. Set the Pot on sauté mode.

5. Add some olive oil and then heat it up and slightly pour the egg mixture. Stir the eggs mixture well.

6. Press the Air Crisp mode and cook the eggs for 15 minutes at 250° Fahrenheit.

7. Portion the omelet into bowls and dollop each bowl with the chopped parsley and peanuts..

Nutrition:

Calories – 257 Protein – 31 g. Fat – 36 g. Carbs – 65 g.

CONCLUSION

Air fryers are a relatively new piece of kitchen gadgetry. They are used by individuals who want to cook healthy foods using less oil and less fat then their conventional counterparts.

In addition to being a healthier alternative to deep frying, air fryers are also fun to use. Air-frying not only produces lots of fun and tasty food, it also saves you time and money. You can cook without the need of a griddle or a stovetop, which frees up your kitchen so you can focus on eating more healthy foods!

It is important to have an air fryer that is up to par. If you want an air fryer that will last for years, make sure that you buy an durable one. To help you choose the right air fryer for you, we have compiled a list of the best air fried ovens! The Airfryer has several seating options. The four different versions include:

Small Seating–The size of the seating area is 13.5" x 8.5" x 9.5".

Medium Seating–The size of the seating area is 20" x 12".

Large Seating–The size of the seating area is 23" x 15".

Extra Large Seating–The size is 32" X 21". The extra large seat could accommodate up to 8 pieces. A small, medium or large fryer is included with every air fryer and can be purchased separately. The only part that may need to be purchased separately is a colander for the basket which will hold up to 16 cups depending on the size of the basket that you are using. There are no other accessories required for the air fryer: please see the specifications on this page for further details.

What's happening to our restaurant food? The answer is rather simple. We are over-cooking and over-frying foods, and most of it is for the wrong reasons.

Nobody wants to eat overcooked, undercooked, or under-salted food. Restaurant owners are turning away good customers in the name of profit.

That's not our fault. It's up to the professional chefs to do a better job with their cooking skills.

We use our Air Fryers to cook foods that don't require cooking at all. We use them to cook and heat our foods in such a way that they're ready to eat right out of the air fryer. There's no need for you to heat up your kitchen with a conventional oven or stove, just put the food in and let it finish fully. You'll be amazed at how delicious your foods can taste when you use an Air Fryer!

Today's busy lifestyle often leaves us with little time to cook. For those of you who don't have time to cook, but still need your food, the air fryer is for you.

An air fryer is an appliance that cooks food by circulating hot air over it. The circulating air causes the food to slowly cook within a sealed container while removing excess oil and fat from the food. By sealing the food in a hermetic chamber during cooking, no additional oil is released into the air. This is important because it prevents the flavor of the food from being compromised. The result is a fast and easy way to prepare delicious meals without having to use any grease or oils while eroding your pantry of oils.

In this air fryer cookbook, we will teach you how to use your air fryer most effectively and how to avoid common mistakes. From learning how to clean and maintain your air fryer to finding creative recipes, this guide will help you get the most out of your air fryer today